INFANTILE PARALYSIS, AND ITS ATTENDANT DEFORMITIES

INFANTILE PARALYSIS, AND ITS ATTENDANT DEFORMITIES

Charles Fayette Taylor

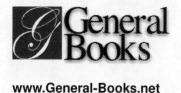

www.General-Books.net

Publication Data:

Title: Infantile Paralysis, and Its Attendant Deformities
Author: Charles Fayette Taylor
Reprinted: 2010, General Books, Memphis, Tennessee, USA
Publisher: Philadelphia, J. B. Lippincott co.
Publication date: 1867
Subjects: Poliomyelitis
Biography Autobiography / General
Health Fitness / Diseases / Nervous System
Medical / Infectious Diseases
Medical / Pediatrics
BISAC subject codes: BIO000000, MED022090, MED069000

INFANTILE PARALYSIS, AND ITS ATTENDANT DEFORMITIES

AND ITS
ATTENDANT DEFORMITIES.
CHARLES FAYETTE TAYLOR, M. D.,
Msident Surgeon New York Orthopedic Dispensary ; Author Of " Me-
Chanical Treatment Op Angular Curvature Of The 8pine ;"
" Spinal Irritation, Or Causes Of Back-ache Among
American Women;" "theory And Practice
Of The Movement-cube," Etc.
PHILADELPHIA:
J. B. LIPPINCOTT and GO.
1867.
Entebbe, According To Act Op Congress, In The Year 1868, Bt CHARLES
FATETTE TAYLOR, In The Clerks Office op The District Court Op The United
States For The Southern District or New York.
Davies and Kent,
Electrotypers and 8/ereotypers, 183 William St. N. Y.
PREFACE.

Notwithstanding the very groat progress made of late years in medicine and surgery, there are still many forms of disease which have not yet received the careful study they require, and about which there is so little to be found in medical literature that the majority of physicians are practically excluded from profiting by the experience of others.

A hundred cases of Infantile Paralysis occurring in the practice of as many diiferent physicians, in different localities, without knowledge of each other, and perhaps each the only case of a lifetime practice, afford,-very imperfect opportunity for that careful, comparative observation which positive science requires. Hence the meagreness of the literature on this subject. Only when some enthusiastic " specialist" calls them from their hiding-places–few in a given locality, but many in community–is there afforded sufficient opportunity for that consecutive and multiplied observation necessary for establishing facts and making deductions. As to the facts set forth in this book, there is scarcely chance for mistake; if the deductions are erroneous, some keener mind will detect the error; but, believing them to be true, the profession have a right to them. I only claim a faithful use of Opportunity, and a careful, honest observation of Pacts.

I wish to express my indebtedness to F. O. Earle M. D., of Chicago, 111., lately assistant in this Institution for the accurate drawings illustrating the text.

If these pages are true, there should be, ten years hence, a smaller proportion of cripples than now distress our sight; and that such may be the case is the fervent hope of

The Author

N. Y. Orthopedic 1303 Bkoadwat cc Institution,)

, Sept., 1866. f

INFANTILE PARALYSIS

ATTENDANT DEFORMITIES.

STATEMENT.

Paralysis in early life is either the direct or remote cause of a large proportion of the distortions of the upper and lower extremities which afflict a certain number in every community.

Perhaps it is not always sufficiently realized that children of a tender age are as much more liable to loss of muscular power than persons of mature age, as they are to any other form of sickness. The young of every kind are always most susceptible and possess least power of endurance, and when not well guarded, suffer most from adverse influences. And this is especially true with regard to affections of the nervous system. Hence there is sufficient reason for the fact, that paralysis is of common occurrence in early life.

DEFINITION.

By the term "Infantile Paralysis" I do not mean simply a paralysis occurring in infancy or childhood; but I desire to restrict the use of the term–and it is so used in this paper–to indicate that form of paralysis which occurs only in infancy. Or if the same form of paralysis be found to occur after maturity, then the term should indicate that which occurs principally and characteristically in children. In fact, as will be hereafter more fully understood, I use the term to express a paralysis peculiar to the growing period. Perhaps, more correctly, it might be called the paralysis of nutrition and development.

FREQUENCY.

There seems to be no doubt that this disease is much more frequent now, and in this coun try, than formerly, and is rapidly increasing. Nor is it difficult to account for this state of things.

PROBABLE CAUSE.

Modern, and especially American, civilization is characterized by peculiar activity of the brain, and this is often carried to great excess.

The motive-force of American progress is brain-power. It is the ceaseless activity of directing mind that, in two centuries, has subdued the wilderness and peopled the continent; that has built vast cities whose commerce reaches the remotest regions of the globe; and that has proved itself capable of solving the most difficult political problems. The creative energy of the distinctively American intellect is recognized everywhere. But such vast results of this creative intelligence have not been accomplished without some sacrifices. It has diminished our physical endurance. As a people, we are dyspeptic, and weak in bodily vigor in the inverse ratio of over-activity of brain. Our laborers have to be imported. We are predisposed to nervous derangements. As a people, we are over-worked. The nervous system becomes exhausted, and a constitution less strong than our own, but more excitable and impressible, is transmitted to our children.

WHY VIGOROUS PARENTS PRODUCE SICKLY OFFSPRING.

It is often asked, "How is it that, when both parents are well and vigorous, the children are often puny and nervous?" The reply must be, that the offspring partake of the parents condition at the time they were begotten. A man who is thoroughly engrossed in business calculations and cares, or even in the pleasures of society, will beget children with physical powers correspondingly subordinated to the nervous. To insure a perfect plant, it is not only requisite that the seed be produced by a strong and vigorous tree, but no drought must have absorbed its sap or untimely frosts have chilled it while the seed was maturing. We have imperfect grapes if an accidental cut lets the juice of the vine leak out.

How, then, can even naturally vigorous persons expect to bear children of equal vigor if begotten while they themselves are exhausted with intense mental labors and excitements? It is a physiological impossibility. Hence our children are born with a surprising degree of nervous irritability; just the temperament for the production of infantile paralysis when favorable circumstances combine to produce it.

MOST COMMON AMONG THE RICH.

And, as may be supposed, this disease occurs most frequently in the families of active business men. Indeed, while strumous diseases abound in the lower classes, I have seen but very few cases of infantile paralysis among them. My whole experience has led me to regard infantile paralysis as being almost confined to the families of active, intelligent men, as above indicated.

ITS PATHOLOGY.

The definite pathology of infantile paratysis is not well understood. I have no theory to offer, and will only assume to present the facts connected with these cases which a pretty extensive, close, and prolonged observation of them may justify me in giving, with a considerable degree of explicitness.

SYMPTOMATOLOGY.

In many cases the paralysis is ushered in with symptoms apparently, in all respects, resembling inflammation of the membranes of the spinal cord. There may be every justification in applying the term spinal or cerebro-spinal meningitis to those cases. But there are many even among these severer cases, where the disturbance follows, rather than precedes, the paralysis, in such a relation as to suggest the i: iquiry, if the disturbance might not possibly have been the effect, rather than the cause of it? So great a shock as the paralyzing of a portion of the body might well be expected to produce a profound impression and serious disturbance.

CONSTITUTIONAL SYMPTOMS SOMETIMES TRIFLING.

There are other cases, however, in which the constitutional symptoms are so trifling, as to tax our minds to account for them in connection with so serious and dangerous a disease as inflammation of the spinal cord or its membranes. Is it possible for distinctive inflammation to be going on in the brain or spinal cord, and the patient exhibit no symptoms which might point to it? And yet there are many cases of infantile paralysis in which there is no noticeable variation from ordinary health, the only symptom to be noticed at the very time, being the paralysis itself.

Casei.–K. GK, at eleven months old, had learned to walk. Suddenly it was observed that she was unable longer to do so, and it was six or eight months later before she regained imperfect locomotive power. The right leg was partially paralyzed; but there was no sickness or other indication of the cause, or even the time of its occurrence. At thirteen I operated on her for partial club-foot.

Case 2.–M. D., though a delicate, nervous child, had no special sickness before or after the paralysis. One day, when two years old, she started to walk across the floor, but became paralyzed when she got to the middle of the room. The paralysis is in the right leg–not complete, though attended with partial arrest of development.

Several other cases of paralysis without constitutional symptoms have come under my observation, though they embrace but a small proportion of the whole. But cases in which the symptoms are very mild are quite common.

In some instances the child is put to bed apparently well, and is found paralyzed in the morning, but without any indication of the time in the night when the paralysis happened, nor was the paralysis followed by any unusual bodily disturbance.

GENERAL HISTORT.

The majority of those cases, however, have about this history: the child is getting its first molar teeth–for the greatest number of cases occur when the child is from fourteen to twenty months old. Sometimes there hns been a diarrhea, or other drain upon the system, or cause of irritation, accompanied with slight fever, though not often enough to keep the child abed. In a few days these symptoms abate and the child appears better; but on making efforts to walk or use his limbs, it is found that he has lost the power to do so. In most cases, the exact time when the paralysis happened is never ascertained.

SELDOM UNCONSCIOUS.

It is seldom that the accession of this form of paralysis is accompanied with unconsciousness. In one case, the child, in apparently perfect health, was sleeping quietly in its cradle, watched fondly by its father. It awoke with a scream, and was found to be completely paralyzed in its entire body. But neither then, nor at any subsequent time, was there any unconsciousness. It is true that there are occasional cases of convulsions followed by infantile paralysis, but there are more cases of convulsions which are not followed by paralysis, and a careful study, when they do exist together, has failed to establish to my mind any direct connection between them. Any sufficient irritation may produce infantile convulsions; but they do not seem to be caused by or to cause the paralysis, though the paralysis may happen at about the same time. As a general rule, this paralysis in young children is accompanied with much less severe symptoms (though this is not always the case) than when the patient is older. With increase of years, the accompanying symptoms in general become more pronounced, and are neither so sudden in their accession, nor do they pass so speedily away. A child from ten to fourteen years old may be sick for several months with a more gradual and less uniform accession of paralysis. This is often accompanied with severe symptoms of what is generally called spinal or cerebro-spinal meningitis.

Infantile apoplexy, with convulsions and paralysis, is quite different from that which we are now considering.

PECULIARITY OF INFANTILE PARALYSIS.

But the form, rather than the origin, of this paralysis is to engage our study.

I wish to call attention to the idea before alluded to, viz., that there is a form of paralysis peculiar to the growing period; that it is most likely to occur at the times of greatest organic or vegetative activity; and that it ceases to act after the organs have attained complete maturity. The periods of life during which it is most liable to occur are from six months to four years of age, and again from ten to fourteen. This form of childhood-paralysis has peculiarities not found in other forms, whether these other forms occur in children or adults. Children as well as adults may have apoplexy, softening, inflammations, blows on the head, etc.; but the resulting paralysis is always essentially different from that which we are now discussing.

NO EVIDENCE OF CENTRAL LESION.

One essential feature of infantile paralysis is. that there is uniformly perfect recovery, so far as we can discover, of whatever disease of the nervous center–if it is ever really caused by a local lesion–which may have caused it.

THE DISEASE PERIPHERIC.

Another essential characteristic of this paralysis is the entire absence of reflex irritability of the muscles, accompanied with a remarkable diminution of capillary circulation in the affected parts, and a correspondingly diminished muscular power. These, and the arrested growth of certain parts, are the only remaining evidence of previous disease. If we can conceive of a general constringing of the capillary vessels, and a shutting off of the capillary circulation, with such a physical condition as would result if the limb had for a long time been tightly bandaged, we should gain a very good idea of the actual condition in infantile paralysis. In fact, my own belief is that the disease is essentially peripheric, and that the great nervous centers are only indirectly and secondarily implicated. On no other hypothesis can I account for all the phenomena of these cases. But whether this suggestion be the true solution or not, the essential condition in infantile paralysis is a cutting off of the capillary circulation and a corresponding loss of muscular irritability; the latter to a great extent, if not wholly, due to this depri vation of blood in the small vessels. And the limb withers as does a plant when the channels to its irrigation are dried up. It is a well-known physiological fact, that the function of any organ is diminished or destroyed by cutting off its supply of blood, and a muscle can no more act without its supply of blood than it can act without the nervous stimulus. In other words, you may paralyze a muscle as completely by stopping its circulation as by dividing its nerve. And it appears to me that the only satisfactory explanation of all the facts in these cases, is to suppose that the paralysis is nearly, if not wholly, due to the diminished capillary circulation rather than, as in other forms of paralysis, to the direct influence of a lesion in the brain or spinal cord. By what precise pathological condition this withdrawing of a large part of the sanguineous fluid is brought about, I have no theory to suggest. There is no doubt as to the fact, however.

TENDENCY TO RECOVERY.

There is another fact of immense importance, and that is, that these cases all tend toward recovery. Very few cases are to be met with where some portions of the originally paralyzed members have not entirely recovered. Of course, there are cases so bad that the sufferer must always remain without hope of essential improvement. Still, the large majority of all the cases I have seen had more than twice the paralysis when it occurred, or when it was first discovered, than they had at the end of the first year. One arm or leg may be paralyzed, but no other portion of the body affected. But more frequently the patient who comes to you a year after the attack, with a single paralyzed arm or leg, was at first paralyzed in both legs or over the whole trunk and extremities, but has recovered except as to some single member. If the recovery is complete, it generally takes place within a few weeks, or at furthest a few months. And it is a curious circumstance, that this spontaneous recovery of a portion of the original paralysis is as much more complete in certain members as it is more imperfect in the remaining ones. That is, in cases of paraplegia for instance, if there is very great improvement or complete recovery in one leg, the other will improve but very little; while, if both legs improve alike, the result will be more general power than in the worse leg, and less power than in the better leg in the first case; as though nature possessed only reserve force enough for the complete recovery of one member, or a less relative improvement if this force be divided between the two. But nature, immediately after such a shock, is seldom capable of repairing the whole damage which has been inflicted. She does with comparative rapidity what she can, and would often do much more if permitted. Many a theory has been triumphantly established by happening to be tried at a time when nature is sure to be using her reserve force to repair damages, and always with more or less success. If the apostles of "electricity," "movements," "strychnia," the "ice bag," etc., have no better data than partial recovery in a few cases within the period of first recuperative effort, their claims rest on a very unsatisfactory basis. I have said in substance, that there is a period of reaction during which time recuperative effort is carried forward with complete, or at least partial success. The partial recovery may be either as to the amount in all affected members, or complete in a portion, while recuperation has but slightly advanced in others apparently no worse originally than the restored portions. But why does the reparative process stop half way? Evidently because nature may have exhausted her reserve force. But why should this reparative effort stop so entirely? Why should we not expect, in accordance with the analogy of all recuperative processes, a continuous, though retarded improvement? While the fact is, that after a certain time improvement is very feebly manifested and very slight in nearly all cases, while in many the condition of the remaining paralyzed limbs actually grows worse as time passes; averaging perhaps one case with another, a total cessation of improvement after the first few months. But I think it can be very clearly established, that when patients do not continue to improve beyond a certain point, or when the improvement is so feeble as only to be recognized from year to year, as well as when there is no longer any improvement to be seen, that it is not always because nature has wholly exhausted herself, but because accidental circumstances have come in to interfere with her work, which would otherwise have gone on much further.

"contractions."

It is noticed that what are called " contractions" of various muscles, accompanied with. heir inevitable results, distortions of joints– begin to appear early in the history of the case. And these so-called contractions go on till the distortions become permanent deformities. When the contractions have proceeded to a certain extent, all increase of muscular power ceases, and the case is generally considered fit only for the orthopedic surgeon. The question arises, "What is the cause of these contractions?" They occur with a preponderance of certain forms; that is, talapes varus is more common than talapes valgus, and contraction of the hamstring muscles are more common than relaxation of the same; but there is the absence of all uniformity or law in reference to it. Certain contractions are most frequent simply because circumstances more frequently favor them than others, and not at all because the disease itself predisposes particular muscles to contract. I have used, and shall continue to use, the word " contractions" in the ordinary way, because the term sufficiently conveys the idea of shortened muscles; but I do not by its use intend to accept the common idea of active contractions of the muscles, in which sense it is generally used.

NO REFLEX CONTRACTION.

It is just here where this form of paralysis differs so radically from all others–from those forms where there is a known lesion in the nerve-center. When there is a rupture and clot in, or inflammation of, the brain or spinal cord or their meninges, the paralysis is always accompanied by reflex movements of the muscles, rigidity, spasm, clonic spasm, pain, numbness, and other indications of disturbance of in-nervation. But in the form of paralysis under consideration–except, possibly, during its in-cipiency–there is a total absence of the least variation of innervation; no difference in the quality or amount of muscular force is ever to be noticed from one day to another, or varying with physical or physiological disturbances. In a word, Infantile Paralysis is peculiar, in that it is characterized by unvarying want of irritability, and this want of irritability is probably the cause of, as well as the extent of, the paralysis. What it is that has deprived the muscles of their irritability, or has deprived the nerves of their power of imparting their stimulus to the muscles; whether the origin was in the nervous centers or in the nervous periphery where the only evidence exists of anything wrong–are questions regarding which I am not prepared to express an opinion. My only object at present is to direct attention to the fact of the unvarying absence of irritability in the muscles themselves, and the want of the ordinary evidence of local disease anywhere in the brain or spinal cord, as the essential characteristic features of this form of paralysis.

SHORTENING OF CERTAIN MUSCLES.

"What, then, causes the muscular contractions, and consequent deformities, which so regularly follow as a seeming necessary consequence of infantile paralysis?" I reply, without hesitation, that contractions and dis tortions are not necessary consequences of this paralysis; and, moreover, that these unhappy results are always and entirely preventable. Indeed, what seem to be contractions of certain muscles–generally the flexors–are not contractions at all, but simply a mechanical shortening of muscles when their attachments are for a length of time brought nearer together. Furthermore, this tendency of muscles to adapt their length to the position in which they are for a time placed, is found to be much less in these cases than where there has been no paralysis at all. And, as might be supposed, the greater the paralysis, the less the shortening of flexor and other habitually relaxed muscles; and, on the other hand, the less the paralysis, the more readily do these muscles assume a permanently shortened condition when the limb is kept for a time in such an attitude that the ends of the muscles approach each other; and when muscles are not paralyzed, they become shortened or elongated according to the accidental position of the limb much more readily than when paralyzed. In case of hip-joint disease, for instance, a very short time will often suffice to cause certain muscles to become so much shortened as to require tenotomy. But in infantile paralysis, the shortening of certain muscles is not the first or principal damage done by improper and careless positions of the paralyzed limbs.

LENGTHENING OF MUSCLES.

The shortening, though the most noticeable, is not the first or worst complication which arises to arrest the progress of improvement and to set in train a series of con- ditions favoring the formation of distortions and deformities. Any position of a limb which allows the extensor muscles to become shortened must inflict a worse damage on the flexors by keeping them extended till they lose their remaining irritability and become degenerated. Now, we have another fact connected with these cases when they have arrived at the stage of deformity, viz., this: the difficulty of treatment consists much less in relaxing the shortened muscles than in giving tone and strength to their antagonists–the lengthened and weakened ones. Indeed, it is this, in the destruction of all remaining muscular irritability, and in many instances the destruction and entire loss of the substance itself of the expanded muscle, which constitutes the principal anxiety in treating this class of deformities. As this important consideration has been many times neglected, if not entirely lost sight of, let us consider the effect of simple extension upon the power and functions of muscular tissue in its healthy state.

Propositions.

In reference to this, the following are believed to be true, viz.: 1st. To retain a healthy muscle in an expanded state for a certain length of time is to diminish or destroy its irritability and contractile force.

2d. To extend a muscle while iu the act of contracting, that is, to overcome it, is to, at once, destroy its irritability and force.

A moments reflection will call up ample illustrations of the correctness of the foregoing statements.

1.–A few months ago, Dr. Win. H. Van Buren read a paper before the New York Academy of Medicine, on the successful treatment of spasm of the sphincter ani, by means of this principle of overcoming muscular action. His treatment for this most distressing disease is as efficacious as it is simple and speedy. By inserting the thumbs within the sphincter and placing the fingers on each haunch as fulcrums, by a powerful effort he stretches the hypertrophied muscle to the fullest extent between the ischii. The irritability and hypertonicity of the sphincter is destroyed and the cure is thus effected. I have seen several cases of relaxed muscles, and one case of real club-foot, which had been caused by a violent extension of muscles while in the act of contracting, which had from that moment caused paralysis of those muscles.

The "india-rubber Man."

" There is a curious illustration of the effect of extension on the ligaments and muscles now in this city. At one of the minor theaters there is exhibiting what is called the "india-rubber man"–an individual whose business it is to contort himself in the most unheard-of and inconceivable manner–dislocating his joints, laying his leg up along the spinal column, and otherwise defying ordinary anatomical laws. How did he attain this remarkable flexibility of joints and relaxation of muscles? Muscles and ligaments are for the purpose of holding the frame together, rather than of facilitating its separation. I have been informed that every day this man subjects himself to a process of continuous stretching of the muscles. A heavy weight is tied to the foot, which he holds pendent, slowly swinging in the air. The same is done to the arms and the whole body. The result is an almost complete destruction of the tonicity of the muscles and a corresponding relaxation of all the tissues. The muscular power is so overcome, and he is so nearly paralyzed, that he can hardly walk; he is wholly incapable of a firm embrace; the spinal column can be made to reverse the natural curves, and, altogether, he is an illustration on a large scale of what must and does occur in a single muscle or group of muscles when subjected to continued or violent traction or extension. The only possible results, loss of irritability and degeneration, are sure to follow. It might be inferred, and such is the fact, that the effect of extension is greater in the paralyzed muscle than in the healthy tissue, and that a slight degree of continuous or comparatively feeble sudden extension, which might be harm- 0 From my paper on "Tenotomy," in the N. Y. State Medical Societys Transactions for 1865.

less in healthy muscles, may be capable of destroying altogether the feeble irritability and power of a recently paralyzed muscle.

"The fact that continuous extension has the power of diminishing, and ultimately destroying, the contractility of muscles, may "be explained without supposing rupture of the fiber-cells, when we remember that the course of the muscular fibrillaa is not straight but zigzag, and that in contraction, this eccentricity is increased, the fibers being thrown up into irregular zigzags. In prolonged extension, these eccentrics may be destroyed and the spaces closed up by the presence and pressure of other straightened-out fibers. Instead of a wavy mass, the fibers may approximate straight lines with a loss of some of the most essential features of muscular tissue and a corresponding loss of contractility.

"It is no doubt already correctly inferred, that I place much more importance on the loss of power in certain muscles as explained above (a relative loss of power beyond the primary effect of the original paralysis), than on the shortened condition of certain other muscles–their antagonists–which is usually referred to as the cause of these deformities."

DIFFERENT DEGREES OF PARALYSIS IN DIFFERENT MUSCLES.

Nothing is more noticeable than the varying degrees of paralysis in different extremities of the same individual, and indeed in the same limb. It is true of these cases, that there may be complete loss of contractility in muscles receiving their nervous supply from the same nerves, and even in contact with other muscles evincing considerable muscular power. There is no other explanation of this apparent defiance of all known physiological laws than the one I have given. But as a matter of fact, these variations–this relative losing or gaining of force–correspond exactly in all cases with the position of the muscles, whether they have been kept in extension or relaxation; for muscles allowed to relax–all other things being equal–gain as much as the extended ones lose. The muscles kept in a shortened position, recover irritability more readily than if kept extended to their natural length; but having no extension, become in time inelastic and tendonous; while those kept unnaturally extended, lose their irritability and become thin and degenerated.

And having thus destroyed the harmonious action of the muscles, as well as their length and mechanical adaptation, we have the first elements of a deformity.

POSITION THE SOLE CAUSE OF SHORTENING AND RELAXATION OF MUSCLES.

Having shown that position of the limbs alone is sufficient to cause deformity even in the healthy subject, it only remains to inquire, "Is this actually the case in infantile paralysis?" The reply must be affirmative.

The particular steps toward the production of deformity subsequent to an attack of infantile paralysis are simple enough. Suppose there is an attack of infantile paralysis during the period of extreme loss of muscular power; the mere weight of the feet is more than the flexors can resist, and they are therefore drawn out. If the patient be abed, the position of the feet is that of extension–the toes droop by their own weight. This dropping down of the foot is aided–if not anticipated and provided against, as it ought to be–by the ordinary handling of the child; the lifting and the friction of the heel against the mattress as the child is placed in bed under the covers; and thus it is kept up till talipes equinus is actually produced.

Fig. 1 represents talipes equinus after the foot has been used in locomotion. And when recovery begins to take place, the first feeble return of contractile power in the flexors is resisted and overcome, while the extensors, already in a shortened position, finding no resistance, assume permanently a shortened position. Now, what is the result from this beginning?

Fig. 1.– Talipes Equinus.

FORMATION OF VARIOUS DEFORMITIES.

The position of the other muscles up to this time may not have been sufficiently unnatural to cause much variation of force in them. But when the patient has regained sufficient strength above the feet to begin to use the legs, he can not use them, because he has no perfect feet to stand on. The destroyed flexors of the feet let the toes drop to the floor, and the shortened extensors hold them there. He is thus forced to sit, unable to make use of the power he has up to this time recovered in the legs above the ankles, because of the deformity of the feet occasioned from want of care, to prevent the relaxation of the gastrocnemii muscles. Not till after the patient begins to sit, do we usually find shortening of the flexors of the legs and thighs. And thus sitting inevitably sets agoing renewed conditions favoring, and if persisted in, compelling, lengthening of the extensors and shortening of the flexors of the legs and thighs. There are seldom other deformities than the simple, equal extension of the flexors of the foot, and shortening of the flexors of the legs and thighs, while the patient remains in bed or only sits. But if he progresses still further, and begins to stand and walk, either the paralysis is so slight that the attitude of standing forces out and lengthens the shortened muscles; and, relaxing the extended ones, allows them to regain their lost power, and the patient recovers more or less perfectly; or, as often happens, the tendo-Achillis will not yield, the patient is thrown off the balance in efforts to sustain himself; the foot is twisted and contorted, and we get variations from talipes equi-nus, which has existed up to this time. The lateral muscles of the foot, already partially overcome by their position, are forced out, as the ankle twists to one side or the other; and we have talipes varus, valgus, and other complications. If but one leg is paralyzed, it is most frequently talipes varus; but if both legs are affected, it is generally talipes varus on the side where the extensors of the knee are weaker, and valgus on the side of the stronger leg. The limping to relieve the weaker leg throws an increased weight on the originally better leg in such a way as to overcome what were and would have remained the stronger muscles, and we have

as a result talipes valgus (see fig. 4), and weakening of the hamstring muscles– results opposite from the first tendency. Fig. 2 very well illustrates this idea. This peculi-

Fig. 2.

arity of locomotion often actually converts

what was, and should have remained, the stronger foot and leg into the more deformed and weaker. For talipes valgus, though not so unsightly, is not so readily cured as talipes varus.

The same general cause may also produce the knock-knee (either alone or in connection with the other deformities), and other complications. So that to cure a talipes varus of one foot, will often go far toward relieving talipes valgus of the other foot. Of course, we may have the same form of talipes of each foot, but then it is usually varus. In general, it may be said that all talipes, except equinus, are produced after the patient begins to bear weight upon his feet, and are caused by the impossibility, in most cases, of standing with shortened tendo-Achillis and talipes equinus. The ankle bends down in the direction of least resistance, which is most frequently outward–

overcoming and elongating the tibialis-anticus and posticus muscles. In other words, talipes varus is the first effort of attempting to stand; while talipes valgus is generally brought on later by walking. But in some cases, placing the child too early on its feet may at once destroy all contractility of the extensors of

Fig. 3.– Talipes Vabus.

the foot, and talipes valgus, or at a later period talipes calcaneus, may be the result.

The last mentioned deformities–talipes valgus and calcaneus–most frequently occur, for the reasons above given, on the least affected leg in paraplegia; or if but one leg is affected, and either of these deformities follows, there is generally less paralysis, except as to the foot, than when followed by equinus or varus. In a word, the limb is strong enough above the ankle to have more weight thrown upon it to support. Fig. 4 represents talipes valgus, and fig. 5 talipes calcaneus.

Fig. 4.– Talipes Valous. Fig. 6.– Talipes Calcaneus.

It is thus seen that these several deformities of the foot–which are often the direct cause of other deformities at a distance from the extremities–are entirely accidental in their origin, the worst form of talipes even occurring on the least paralyzed leg; the paralysis being the occasion, but not the direct cause, of these deformities. I have dwelt on the manner in which club-foot is produced in these cases, because it is the first to appear, and is the most conspicuous. The other distortions of the limbs come on later, because the conditions favoring their production are less constant and are generally entirely wanting for a long time after the accession of the paralysis; being deferred often till after the deformities of the foot have become a fact largely influencing the formation of the other distortions. As the patient recovers, if he can not walk, or walks with great effort and imperfectly, he must sit a great part of the time. Hence, after a while, shortening of the flexors of the thigh and leg begins to be manifest, with the inevitable relative diminution of irritability and strength, and finally degeneration of the quadriceps extensor of the leg and even the glutei. It does not take but a slight flexion at the several joints to cause a deviation from the equilibrium and the throwing of the osseous framework off its balance, when the whole weight is thrown on the muscles and ligaments. These give way in various directions, producing a sad catalogue of deformities.

THESE DEFORMITIES AEE ALWAYS PREVENTABLE.

If I have stated nothing but the facts–and I have simply told my experience, begun with no theory and anticipating no conclusions–it follows as an inevitable corollary, that the deformities ordinarily attending infantile paralysis are entirely preventable! I do not say that the paralysis itself is always curable; but, that the distortions generally following it are not a necessary consequence of the paralysis, and need not exist with it; and they will not exist if seasonable and proper precautions are taken to avoid the secondary injuries to which the peculiar condition of the muscles renders them liable. In these cases no muscles contract; they only become shortened after having been kept relaxed for a considerable time. The improvement, be it more or less, would be uniform if the flexors of the foot and extensors of the leg and thigh were not kept in an extended position till they had lost their irritability and force. If the feeble muscles and ligaments of the joints were not subjected to overwhelming strain, by bearing too early an injudicious weight, they would not give way under the first attempt at exercise, instead of being strengthened by it–which they might be, if proper precaution were observed,

TREATMENT OF THE PARALYSIS.

The treatment of infantile paralysis in the early stages consists, for the most part, in noninterference with the recuperative efforts of nature. While the nervous system is completely overwhelmed by a recent shock, no treatment (for the paralysis) is good treat ment. The general indications of the case should first be attended to, of course. For many months, and till interrupted by the causes heretofore named, the tendency is toward recovery; though this recovery is, or seldom would be, complete without appropriate aid, and not often even then. Still, as I have said, the natural tendency is toward recovery; and let no one fancy that his pet remedy administered at this stage has effected the change for the better. He may deceive himself, but not those who have had experience in these cases.

We are to remember how little it may take to injure the enfeebled muscular tissue, and diligently guard the patient from possible harm–knowing the direction from which injury is most likely to come. To this end, first of all, the patient should have the feet protected from extension by their own weight. This can be effectually done by placing them on a kind of sandal or shoe, as shown in fig. 6, for keeping the foot at a right-angle with tlie leg. A careful decumbency is sufficient for other muscles while the patient remains in bed. After a time, the reaction from the first prostration begins to take place, the febrile symptoms subside, and all the bodily functions resume their usually healthful course, except the power of motion in certain extremities. Even here, there is generally some decided improvement. If one extremity continue paralyzed, others, which at first seemed to be equally affected, rapidly regain their usual strength. But in certain members, the progress of amelioration is slow, and, may-be, not sufficient to be noticed under ordinary circumstances.

RECUPERATIVE PERIOD.

And here we arrive at a very critical period. A certain amount of recuperation has taken place with a corresponding amount of improvement in some, at least, of the muscles. How shall we keep up this recuperative process? Every organ is strengthened by the proper exercise of its function. Whatever power there may be in a muscle after a certain time, needs to be used in order to develop more. But there may not be enough for the purposes of locomotion or actual bodily use; and to let what has accumulated remain inactive, is to enfeeble what force there is for want of use. On the one hand, there is the danger of breaking down the inadequate muscles by placing the whole weight of the body on them in premature efforts to walk; and on the other hand, without effort the muscular strength will not continue to increase.

LEGITIMATE MUSCULAR ACTION.

Evidently, then, we must contrive to afford the muscles opportunity to act within their capacity–alike avoiding inactivity or over-action–until their development has reached the point where they are capable of being made available in sustaining the weight of the body, and in locomotion. The muscles of a leg, for instance, may be capable of sustaining thirty pounds weight, not only without injury, but with actual benefit; when sixty pounds–the weight of the patient, perhaps–would cause it to break down. There is evidently. then, but one thing to do in such a case. We must furnish tlie muscle an exercise that shall not exceed its capacity. If thirty pounds be the extent of its force, thirty pounds must be the extent of its exercise. And not until the powers of the muscles have been developed, till they are equal to sustaining the weight of the body, should they be required to sustain it. There is no physiological principle more clear or simple. The leg of a paralyzed child in relation to its body may be compared to those of an infant called upon to support the trunk of a man; they can not do it, and should not be allowed to attempt it till they liave grown equal to their load. But every particle of latent force calls for use; action is its life and growth; and under these unusual circumstances we are called upon to furnish the opportunity for whatever force there is, to act.

MUSCULAR DYNAMOMETERS.

This involves contrivances for the display and use of small amounts of muscular force; to specimens of which the attention is now invited. These muscular dynamometers–for such they properly are–embrace the principle of local exercise, which is equivalent to a great saving of force, in having it under control and direction– as well as the one more particularly under consideration, viz.: the ability to detect and use minute–and without such facilities inappreciable–quan- titles of muscular power. Fig. 7, for exercising the flexors and extensors of the feet, is contrived on the principle of a balance; when

Fig. 7.

the weight, W, is moved to one side or the other of the center, in the slightest degree, the force is opposed to the flexors or extensors of the foot; and instead of supporting the whole weight of the body above, only a few ounces may oppose the muscles.

Figs. 8 and 9 represent contrivances on the same principle, but adapted to attain the same purposes with reference to the flexors and extensors of the leg. They all are reversible and unlimitedly adjustable. As the mechanical action of the different parts

Fig. 8.

of our locomotive apparatus varies at each joint, each contrivance must be adapted to its special needs. But the principle of making them all measures of force, and the means for using and developing the same, must remain the same throughout all. In the apparatus represented in fig. 10 the whole leg is used

as in the very act of walking, but with any desired amount of force, from a few ounces up to more than the weight of the humun

Fig. 9.

form; and the contrivance is so arranged that as the limb is flexed the resistance is less, which increases as the limb is extended and stronger, so as to secure a steady, equal amount of effort in all positions; the resistance being more when the leg is extended and stronger, and less when the leg is flexed and weaker. And so every apparatus for

Fig. 10.

giving exercise to a part must be adapted to the special mechanical arrangement of the member. If the patient has been carefully attended, so that no damage has been done by faulty positions while in a state of muscular atony, there will be no difference in the rate of recovery, nor will there be shortening or lengthening of different muscles, and the patient can begin to stand and walk at a much earlier stage, and with much less strength, than when a very small amount of shortening of muscles has been allowed to take place. The reason for this is, that the least contraction of the flexor muscles will at once throw the patient out of his natural erect position, and the weight of the body must be held entirely by force of the muscles instead of resting on the bony framework, with only sufficient muscular aid to keep it erect. In other words, every joint will be slightly flexed with an impossibility of complete extension. If these "contractions" have already begun, the first attention must be paid to removing them; and when they are re-cent and slight, extension of all the joints may be made, and the patient assisted to keep in the standing position by an apparatus represented in fig. 11. The move-able handles, C C, with the pad against the knees at A, controlled either by the patient or another, makes forcible or allows muscular extension at will. The position itself—when not obtained by too much effort—is of considerable value in aiding development. The simple, upright position, even when main-

Fig. 11.

tained without the aid of the muscles, seems to determine a certain amount of blood into the lower extremities–perhaps by gravity–to their decided benefit. And this leads us, by a natural step, to consider here the importance of securing as complete a circulation in the paralyzed members as can possibly be obtained. It was observed in the first part of this paper, that the special peculiarity of infantile paralysis was that it was characterized by a greatly diminished capillary circulation, making the loss of function due, at least to a certain degree, to this cause.

THERAPEUTIC VALUE OF WARMTH.

All those who have had experience in these cases have recommended the warm or hot local bath as of great value. My experience is, that the value of local heat in these cases can not be over-estimated. It is a constant experience, that a limb which shows no sign of motion before, will generally give good evidence of awakened vitality after it has been immersed in a hot bath. It is an almost daily occurrence, that muscles which have remained for years, apparently, without power of motion, will evince contractile effort after the blood has been called into the inter-muscular capillaries by a high degree of heat. My plan is to apply the heat daily before beginning their exercises; and in the first stages of the disease, the affected limbs should be kept not merely warm but actaally hot, by means of heated bricks, bottles of hot water, etc. But a dry heat is very much better than the moist heat of a water bath. Moisture not only can not be borne at so high a temperature as dry heat, but it soaks the epidermis, making the skin sensitive, and preventing frequent repetitions; once a day is all it can usually be administered. And, also, a large portion of the heat imparted by the water bath is carried off again in the subsequent evaporation from the surface and epidermis into which it has been absorbed. But a dry heat can be continued for hours and repeated at short intervals, besides being carried to a much higher degree. Parents are directed to prepare a screen large enough to protect the whole body of the child. This is put before the fire, and the patient is placed behind it. Its legs are thrust through and placed on a bench very near the fire, where they are kept for hours at a time. The heat should be kept from the childs head and trunk, as we want not only positively but relatively high heat. A still more effective plan is to place a gas-stove in a wooden box, one side of which is curtained with a piece of cloth having holes, through which the feet and legs are thrust into the box, where they are subjected to any degree of temperature desired. Nothing can be more easily regulated or more simple in its operation.

NECESSITY FOR EARLY AND CAREFUL MANAGEMENT.

It is believed that if infantile paralysis were managed in its first stages on the plan above indicated, having in view the physiological indications and aiming at ultimate good results, there would be a much larger percentage of recoveries than at present. My own cases–those in which I have had the good fortune to see them soon after the attack–have uniformly disappointed every one in the amount of their recovery.

Case 3.–A single case will illustrate the principle. C. H. 0., of Indiana, a lad ten years old, was brought to me in June, 1862, with paralysis of both lower extremities. The attack had only been five weeks previously, and though it was a severe case, it gave me another desirable opportunity of conducting a case from very near the first according to my own ideas of treatment. The lad was large, active, intelligent– a usual characteristic in these cases–particularly precocious, with a rather slender physical organization. About five weeks before, on occasion of what was supposed to have been slight over-exertion, he was taken with symptoms usual with this kind of paralysis. There were a few days of febrile disturbance, which at first it was difficult to account for, but when the paralysis was discovered, was called spinal meningitis. But whatever the cause, his bodily health was perfect when I saw him, and he had been brought a thousand miles to me without the least inconvenience. There was slight motion in the lower extremities, but utter inability to walk or stand; the legs were diminished in size and lower in temperature than natural; all the other functions were perfectly performed; almost better, his parents thought, so far as appetite, digestion, and flow of animal spirits were concerned, thau before the attack. His treatment was conducted on the principles and substantially after the plan set forth in the preceding pages. As he could not walk, he used to slide himself along upon his haunches by his hands, and it was fully two years before he could walk alone. But he did walk at last; and for the past two years there has not been found a more active and enduring young person of his age and constitution in his native city (Richmond, Ind.) There is no dropping of the foot, twisting of the ankle, weakness of the knees, or halt or limp to show that for two years and over he was paralyzed and not able to take a step! But the point I wish to make in bringing this case forward is, that during all these two years of paralysis there were no so-called "contractions" with their attendant distortions and deformities of the paralyzed lower extremities! If deformities are a necessary consequence of this form of paralysis, why did they not occur in this case? They were not removed–had they been, the recovery would never have been perfect; but they were prevented, by not allowing the conditions to occur which cause shortening of the muscles. Then why not prevent them in au cases? I do not hesitate to say that I believe they might be thus prevented in all cases; though I do not pretend that even to prevent deformity would in all cases be followed by complete recovery from the paralysis, though it would certainly increase the number of recoveries.

INJURY FROM DELAY.

But it unfortunately happens that in the greater number of instances the orthopaedic surgeon does not see the case in the early stage of the disease, when he might advise a course calculated to prevent deformity and give the greatest chance of ultimate recovery; but the patient is brought to him with not only paralysis, but paralysis accompanied with different forms of distortions of the affected limbs. He is not permitted to cure the case now, even if a cure at first had been possible; but he must address himself to the removing, so far as possible, of the two-fold damage. It is now too late to think of radical cure; hereafter he must labor long and anxiously to imperfectly repair what might have been much more easily prevented. But the slightest improvement in a child or young person who is to enjoy such improvement for a lifetime is to be diligently sought and gratefully acknowledged.

TREATMENT OF THE DEFORMITIES.

We come now to the means for removing the deformities allowed to be attendant on infantile paralysis. And even here the deformity itself is not that which is the chief thought; for although there is something very tangible in a club-foot, our surgery should come in to divide the shortened tendon for an ulterior object, the relieving and restoration of the flexor muscles. Our tenotomy should have quite as much reference to the lengthened as to the shortened muscles. And this is the secret—which should be no secret—of the frequent failure of tenotomy to effect that permanent benefit which it at first promised and seemed to afford. When no attention is given to the development of the antagonists of the shortened muscles, there is always danger of a recurrence of the same condition. It must occur again if the same causes continue to exist after, as before, the operations. Where there is but partial paralysis, and the shortening not extreme— implying retention of a certain amount of force in their antagonist muscles—there may be spontaneous development of these weakened but not wholly exhausted muscles occurring too soon after tenotomy to allow of ultimate! losing what is gained. But here, as in all cases, the tenotomy was but the first step—the loosening of the cords which prevented motion, and the development—which is the real cure—followed as a natural consequence. So that while our art of surgery or mechanics is applied directly to the tendons and muscles which resist the movements and bind up the parts in a distorted position, the real result—which does not make, but permits the cure—is the releasing the drawn out and weakened muscles. There are indeed instances when we are content to accept much less; where, if the limb be straightened, that is all we hope to do. In such a case, the lower part of the leg is used by active muscles higher up, for purposes of locomotion, the same as a wooden leg would be, and it has precisely the same use; it is the bony frame, not the muscles, which is used.

Observing that patients with paraplegia differed exceedingly in the apparent use of their legs—some with what seemed much greater paralysis appearing to surpass in powers of locomotion those retaining considerable muscular force—I was for a long time at a loss to account for this singular state of things. But it seems to be the fact, that where the paralysis is very complete, little or no shortening of the muscles takes place—as from the nature of the case we might on reflection see must be the fact—and the whole limb, or that part of it below the knee, is moved by the muscles attached to the trunk, which always retain much greater force—as an artificial limb would be. And if the leg and thigh are in the same perpendicular line, the weight of the body is easily borne on the osseous framework without the help of the muscles; and, unless the toe is hit, or some cause should throw the knee forward, the patient can progress without much trouble. The foot is thrown far forward with a peculiar swing—especially peculiar when both legs are in this condition–and brought slightly back, and the knee pressed backward by leaning forward the trunk, so as to be sure that the knee-joint is fully extended. In general, the person has so often pressed the knee backward with the hand on rising from a chair and in other situations when he did not feel secure on his feet, that the posterior ligaments have been stretched till the leg no longer forms a perpendicular line, but curves backward. This enables him to make very good locomotion; but it effectually prevents the slightest improvement in the power of the muscles after the moment the knee passes back of the perpendicular line of the leg.

NECESSITY FOR CARE AND JUDGMENT IN THE USE OF MECHANICAL FORCE.

The flexor muscles are extended and weakened by extreme extension, and the extensors are never excited to action–the motion at the knee, in such a case, being a mechanical one, effected by flexors of the thigh; and hence they become degenerated for want of use. The same cause produces precisely the same result in the non-paralyzed muscles, as the following case will illustrate:

Case 4.–A young girl had been treated for morbus coxarius by counter-extension. The treatment had been successful so far as to arrest the diseased action in the hip-joint; but when she attempted to walk, it was found that she had almost no strength in the knee, and in that condition I first saw her. I found, on examination, both extensors and flexors of the leg with nearly complete paralysis, and so great relaxation of the posterior ligament and flexor muscles of the knee, that on extension the knee would be pressed some three inches back of the natural position. Hence the injury by severe extension of the flexors and degeneration and atrophy from non-use of the extensors of the leg, precisely as so often happens in infantile paralysis. It was ascertained, on inquiry, that, in effecting the counter-extension for relieving the hip-joint, the adhesive straps had been applied to the leg entirely below the knee, the attending physician apparently not suspecting that a force which could overcome the powerful muscles about the hip-joint would be liable to draw asunder the weaker muscles of the knee. This case did not, and could not, recover without aid, while the leg was used, because it was, from the nature of the case, self-continuing. It was cured by the same means employed for the same condition when preceded by infantile paralysis. This treatment consists simply in applying an apparatus with a stop-joint at the knee, which will entirely prevent excessive extension, or, indeed, will not allow the extension to be quite as complete as natural. If the apparatus is so adjusted that in standing the knee can not quite reach the perpendicular, that situation greatly stimulates the extensor muscles, which soon recover when there has been no paralysis; and more slowly, of course, if the muscles have been previously paralyzed. The flexors also, kept continuously relaxed, soon begin to shorten according to the general law in such cases.

INFLUENCE OF DIVERSE CAUSES.

But this deformity (that produced by extension) is less frequent than permanent flexion at the knee; and when it does happen, it can nearly always be traced to the effects of oft-recurring over-straining, rather than to constant position. For instance, the talipes varus and flexion at the knee of one leg, which is originally the leg the more paralyzed, may cause talipes valgus and extreme extension at the knee on the other leg, which was originally but slightly affected, and would have entirely recovered but for these accidents. I say accidents, because it is owing to the crippled condition of the one leg that the weight of the body is constantly thrown over upon the better leg in such a manner as to overcome the recovering, though still enfeebled muscles of the other. Thus we have produced talipes valgus by the extension of the peronei and gastrocnemius muscles. At the same time we may have knock-knee, or extreme extension of knee by relaxation of internal or posterior ligaments, as shown in fig. 2.

This explains why we so generally find such strange disproportions in the location and degrees of weakness in different groups of muscles. There is no deformity, however anomalous it may seem, that can not be accounted for in the operation of wholly preventable causes.

We find on the side of weaker gluteii the stronger flexors; and as we examine each set of muscles which acts in concert with others to produce a certain motion, there is never the same condition in the corresponding group of muscles in the two legs, nor in those co-operating to produce combined movements in the same leg; this result having been produced by the purely accidental causes just explained.

EXTENSION–TENOTOMY.

In case there is flexion at the knee (fig. 12), even when it is only slight, if the

Fig. 12.

strength of the muscles has been so weakened, either by the previous paralysis or by subsequent persistent extension of the ex tensor muscles as to be unable to support the body, no attempt at developing these muscles will be at all availing until they have been liberated from their unnaturally drawn out position. This may be done either by dividing the tendons of the shortened flexor muscles or by extending them by mechanical means, when that is possible. In either case, and in all such cases, the object is to liberate the confined joint and allow of motion, in order that development, which has been stopped, may go on. In many cases it will not be found necessary to use the knife. But when tenotomy is resorted to, some contrivance for keeping up extension will be found absolutely necessary, in order to sustain the limb in the extended position until all the parts have become adapted to their changed position. Experience had taught me this. I noticed, as previously remarked, that persons with the knee bending slightly backward could walk, bearing their weight upon the leg, though there was little or no muscular power; while a very slight flexion at the knee was always attended with utter useless-ness of the leg in spite of considerable power in the muscles. After vain efforts to develop sufficient force in the extensor muscles to sustain the body, I proposed to convert the forward into a backward bending at the knee, and adopted. an apparatus (fig. 12) for that purpose. The difficulty of canying the plan into successful execution did not depend so much on the resistance of the muscles as on the altered form of the knee-joint itself. After the posterior portions of the articulations have been in contact for a number of years, they become so altered that when weight is placed on the leg, the knee springs forward from the mere shape of the joint itself. This caused the necessity for a prolonged use of the apparatus with the idea of continuing the contact of the anterior portions of the joint until time and use had so modified them that this difficulty should be removed. As the ultimate object was to force extension so far that the knee should pass back of the perpendicular, the action of the apparatus was kept up in several cases for six months, and in a few cases even longer than that. The patients, rejoicing in the ability to use the leg–which they could on wearing the apparatus–and dispense with crutches, were careful to secure adequate support by keeping up extension.

RELAXATION OF EXTENDED MUSCLES CAUSES A RESTORATION OF IRRITABILITY.

What was my astonishment and delight to find, in all cases, after a lapse of a few months, that the same extensor muscle which had before exhibited no power, had regained considerable contractility from having been kept a long time in merely a relaxed position! However, this corresponds with other related facts in connection with these cases. But this fact alone, viz., the ability to restore, partially at least, an enfeebled muscle by persistently relaxing it, is of great consequence in the treatment and prognosis of these unfortunate cases.

This history would not be complete without this concluding experience.

Case 5.–One patient–a boy–had progressed so far that he began to show considerable power of extension at the knee, and could even take a few steps without the aid of his apparatus or crutch, when one of my associates, during my absence, made him an instrument, like many used, allowing "a little motion" at the knee, with the not unnatural idea of "exercising the muscles." At each step there was a slight flexion at the knee and downward movement of the whole body, as its weight would overcome the muscles. The result was, much to his chagrin, that less than two months of this kind of "development" sufficed to destroy every vestige of power which the quadriceps extensor had previously acquired! A return to the former treatment again restored the muscle to its former condition, and a continuance of the treatment secured a continuance of improvement. The corollary to such experience is, that any " motion" which allows a muscle to be overcome is injurious to its contractile power. A muscle knows no other motion" than that which allows it to Contract !

APPLIANCES CONSTRUCTED ON FALSE PRINCIPLES.

It follows, then, that all those appliances with elastic straps, ostensibly to give exercise to the muscles, but really allowing them to be overcome with a part, instead of the whole weight of the body–a difference which the muscles, so long as they are still overcome, must fail to appreciate–must be wrong in principle. If the springs are stiff enough to sustain the weight, then there might as well be no springs at all. Adjustable stop-joints are better. The apparatus for extension at the knee is simply a stop-joint with a screw and knee-cap, as shown in the cut (fig. 12). But the extension must be unvaryingly persisted in till the ultimate object is reached.

UNEQUAL ATROPHY OF DIFFERENT MUSCLES NOT CAUSED BY THE PARALYSIS.

It must be seen that the variations in the relative strength, as well as the length of different muscles, do not depend on causes existing in the muscles themselves, or even on any peculiar condition of the nervous system or the nervous centers. As another illustration of the manner in which muscles may be injured by remote causes, take the following, which embraces a large class. Cases often occur like this: a child is attacked with infantile paralysis, and recovers, or is supposed to have recovered. But in a few years it is noticed that there is a peculiarity about the gait; the child walks well enough on level ground, but is apt to stumble in rough places, and finally it is perceived that the leg is growing small above the knee!

INFLUENCE OF DISTANT CONTRACTIONS ON THE PHYSICAL MECHANISM.

Examination reveals a slight shortening of the tendo-Achillis; the heel does not quite touch the floor in walking, and there is complete paralysis and atrophy of the quadriceps extensor of the leg. The fact is, that while the original paraljsis lasted, a slight shortening of the extensor muscles of the foot had taken place–just enough to cause the ball of the foot to touch the ground before the heel–and a very little talipes equinus was the result. Actiag as a lever, of which the ball of the foot forms one arm, the leg has been extended by the weight upon it without the aid of the quadriceps extensor. At every step the toes reached the ground first, and the knee is literally drawn backward by the tendo-Achillis, while the extensors of the leg are not allowed to act at all. The result is, that in process of time these extensor muscles become completely powerless and degenerated from want of use. Those muscles are, much worse than if the paralysis had been somewhat greater; for, in that case, the talipes equinus would have been severe, or have been converted into a talipes varus, and in either case, by weakening the ankle, the backward action of the tendo-Achillis is lost, and the extensors of the leg would be obliged to act. As these cases–which are not rare–can walk well on ordinary ground, and only fail in certain situations; and as the slight elongation of the foot just about compensates for the shortening in other locations, it is sometimes difficult to make the parents understand that the case can be cured only by making it temporarily appear worse.

EQUALIZING MUSCULAR AND MECHANICAL POWER.

For the first step is to lengthen–which is to weaken–the tendo-Achillis; but this at once deprives the leg of its power of mechanical extension at the knee until those extensors shall be increased in power sufficient to perform their legitimate functions. The heel is let down–the leg is thus slightly shortened–so that, altogether, for several months there will be exhibited increased weakness and halting. But it is the only road to restoration, for if not counteracted there is danger of gradual increase of malpositions and ultimate permanent lameness.

To treat a case of this kind, if it be severe, the tendon may be divided; but generally, if the shortening is not great, it can be overcome by an apparatus for producing extension of the tendo-Achillis, worn at night ouly, but persisted in for months, and made to act very efficiently. (See fig. 11.) Of course, in connection with shortening of the tendo-Achillis there is always more or less feeble-nejss of the flexors of the foot. I remember several cases when, after consultation, the parties were sent home with no other advice than to keep up nightly extension with the simple apparatus with which they were provided, when they returned after a number of months with very tolerable restoration of power in both extensors of the knee and flexors of the foot. But they must have the plan of treatment fully explained to them, and must also be of the most intelligent class, as it will be found difficult to make them pursue a treatment which, at first, causes the patient to be more lame and to appear worse from day to day. But it will be found that as the vicarious extension decreases, the legitimate action of the true extensors of the leg will be stimulated, and in most cases the best result attained.

I should say that it must be a very mild and simple case where extension during the night alone will suffice to lengthen the shortened muscles or allow the elongated flexors to contract. In most cases, an apparatus with a flexion screw, as shown at the ankle in fig. 12, is worn during the day; and if the case is very bad, the same may be used at night also. Whatever the means, they must be made efficient.

TREATMENT OF TALIPES.

With regard to the treatment of the different forms of club-foot which so generally are allowed to follow infantile paralysis, the same principle of treatment should be adopted as in distortions of other joints; we extend or divide the shortened tendons in order to relieve extended and weakened muscles; and we liberate the confined joints in order that motion and development may take place. The only difference between these deformities of the feet and those occurring in other localities consists in their more complex nature, and consequently in the greater difficulty of adapting apparatus to the accomplishment of several different and distinct ends at the same time. But this task need not be so difficult as it is often made.

When it is once understood that talipes equinus is the first, and simplest, and most natural sequence of the paralysis–the weight of the foot being all that is necessary to produce it–and that no other form of talipes is likely to occur while the patient lies in bed; and, moreover, that the bending of the ankle outward (varus) is the result of weight on a foot with a shortened tendo-Achillis; and that bending inward (valgus) of the ankle is the result of weight partially overcoming the gastrocnemius, soleus, etc.; and talipes calcaneus of weight entirely overcoming those muscles, it will be found that the nature and treatment of these deformities are capable of great simplification. (See figs. 1, 3, 4, and 5.) I have not alluded to the adductors and abductors of the foot– the tibiales anticus and posticus, and the peronei, because I believe their influence so exceedingly small in the formation of talipes that they need not necessarily be taken into account; though once formed they exert a minor influence in maintaining the deformity. In talipes equi-nus and varus (figs. 1 and 3), the tendo-Achillis is shortened; in talipes valgus and calcaneus (figs. 4 and 5), the tendo-Achillis is lengthened. On the other hand, the flexor muscles . J of the foot are extended and powerless in talipes equinus and varus, and are shortened and active in talipes valgus and calcaneus. The production of the valgus and varus, though overcoming the internal or external lateral ligaments of the ankle and the peronei or tibiales muscles, as the case may be, must have either extension or shortening of the tendo-Achillis as a condition precedent. The extreme distortion of the foot itself, with the great alteration in form of the tarsal bones in some cases, are all secondary and subordinate matters, and disappear gradually when the causes producing them are reversed in time. The one essential fact which preponderates in considering the principle to be kept in view in adapting apparatus to overcome these distortions–for every apparatus should be the exponent of an idea–is that the os colds is the point which determines and hence controls talipes! Without a shortening or lengthening of the tendo-Achillis there could scarcely be a club-foot. And while we have to provide for all the sequences of these primary conditions, yet it should never be lost sight of, that the cause must be removed before the cure can be considered complete.

APPARATUS FOE TALIPES.

The apparatus which I have used for several years with great satisfaction, consists of a "night" shoe and a "day" shoe. The former is also worn during the day when the patient can not walk, and the latter is often worn at night instead of the night shoe. The first consists simply of two pieces of thin board–one for the sole of the foot, and the other and longer piece to pass up the back of the leg nearly to the knee. The rest consists of the various straps and the way in which they are adjusted. Much of the inefficiency of many of the shoes for club-foot arises from the defective manner of applying the straps. For instance, how can a strap which passes over the instep be expected to resist the strength of the gastrocnemius, soleus, etc.? Even after tenotomy, the pressure on the top of the foot is often unbearable, besides impeding the circulation. A better way is to pass the strap entirely around the

Fig. 13.

ankle (fig. 13), fastening it on the same side from which it started. Thus, in fig. 13, the gtraps, B B, start at the heel and pass above the os calcis around the ankle, just under the malleolus, and fasten on the same side and about three inches from the point they started from. The straps pass around the ankle in opposite directions. It will be seen that these straps, instead of pressing on a surface of only an inch or two in front of the foot, have their pressure distributed over more than the entire distance around the ankle. They also pass above the heel; and besides firmly holding the ankle, they make direct traction on the tendo-Achillis by their downward action on the os calcis. By tightening the straps, C C, the extensor muscles are effectually antagonized. The strap A simply holds the top of the apparatus in place. This apparatus is just as effectual in either of the other forms of club-foot as in the variety just mentioned, all necessary variation of action being secured by a slight variation in the application of the straps. For instance, by placing the foot piece in contact with the sole of the foot, and allowing the leg piece to pass under the leg, as shown in the cuts, figs. 14 and 15, one strap, B B, is passed around the ankle, which is turned out as before, while the other, A A, is passed around the os calcis to act in the opposite direction; while a third, C, holds the meta-tarsis in the same direction that the strap A A holds the os calcis. Now, if we draw

Fig. 14.

the strap D, the leg piece is drawn under the leg, and we have secured a most effectual and complete lateral action without the use of a spring or joint. If we now tighten the strap E (fig. 15), as in talipes equinus, we have effectually antagonized both the lateral and posterior muscles, and have also the quality and degree of action entirely within our control. It is obvious that the same

Fig. 15.

apparatus will apply equally well to talipes valgus or varus, by simply reversing the action of the straps. For talipes calcaneus it is only necessary to supply the posterior strap, C (fig. 1C), to make it a complete relief to the extensors of the foot and an antagonizer of the flexors.

When these cases are taken at or near their early stages, especially before the tarsal bones have been subjected to the weight

Fig. 16.

consequent to walking, it only requires perseverance to accomplish a restoration of the equipoise between the different sets of muscles; and this can generally be done without dividing them. But in long-standing cases we meet with great difficulty in the alterations and misplacements of the tarsal bones. In all such cases we are obliged to keep up the support, not only till relaxation of some, and retraction of other muscles, has restored a harmony of action, but also till the osseous structures have been brought back, by constant pressure in the right direction, to a natural shape and position. In this case the appliances just described, as they act principally on the muscles, would not be sufficient. We must use the same weight which was instrumental in forcing the osseous structures out of shape and position to bring them back again. The patient must walk; and while walking he must have such appliances as shall not merely allow him to progress, but shall also convert what formerly was the means of forcing the tarsal bones out of shape, into the means of forcing them back to their proper position. No apparatus without a lateral action can do this. With a lateral deformity in talipes varus and valgus, it is necessary to meet, check, and reverse this tendency by lateral antagonism. The ankle brace represented in fig. 17 is calculated to meet the indications in such cases. It consists of a T-shaped piece of steel, 0, with the lower end

Fig. 17.

bent at right angles and passing under the sole of the shoe to which it is fastened. The cross piece is just below the malleolus, and from each end a strap, D D, passes around the ankle. Around the heel, but acting in the opposite direction, is the strap A, one end of which is fastened into the sole of the shoe, and the other, after passing around the heel, goes through the back of the shoe and is received by the slit, B, in the end of the curved steel piece, which is a continuation of C. At G is a joint allowing flexion and extension, and at H is a stop-joint regulated by a screw, I, which completely controls the lateral action of the joint. It will be seen that, as the straps D D and B B act in opposite directions, either by drawing these straps, or by the screw, I, we have the power of turning the ankle outward or inward at pleasure, and can convert the tendency to a talipes varus into that for talipes valgus, or the reverse, at once. As a practical matter, it takes much time and perseverance, careful attention, and a nice adjustment to keep the apparatus constantly in order till the form of the foot has been changed. The whole weight of the body resting on the apparatus, and the distortion being resisted by it, it must be made exceedingly strong. It is never best to sacrifice efficiency to lightness.

THE OS CALCIS.

It will be seen that in all these appliances the os calcis may almost be considered as the helm by which the position of the foot is controlled. And when the correct position of this bone is secured and maintained a sufficient length of time, the other distortions of the tarsus will sooner or later disappear.

CONDITION REQUISITE IN APPARATUS.

Thus far I have spoken only of the mechanical appliances which seem best to answer indications in the support of feeble joints; to counteract the effect of shortened muscles, and to relieve those whose position was destructive to their irritability and force. The main idea in these contrivances was to have them accurately meet the indications–whether of extension, relief, or support –and to see that they interfered with no other functions than those they were intended to aid or resist. Adjustability and efficiency must always be the grand object in the use of mechanical agencies. There must always be a principle of treatment which should be as closely followed in the use of mechanical, as in the use of any other therapeutic means.

DEVELOPMENT, THE PRINCIPAL OBJECT.

But even in these severe cases, when paralysis, time, and neglect of suitable preventive means have done their worst, we should still be actuated by the same idea in the hope of securing the largest amount of muscular development of which the case is capable. Although the mechanical treatment does secure advantages of its own, it arises from the fact that, by removing obstructions and protecting the distorted members from injury while using them, there is a certain amount of spontaneous development. This spontaneous development often, and in mild cases generally, amounts to sufficient to complete the cure. But even in these cases the use of apparatus only prepares the way, by removing obstructions, to the natural position of the parts, and allowing a natural action of the muscles. Development or increase of muscular power is the only source of lasting improvement after all. For, no matter how much or how often these distortions are overcome, either by surgical or mechanical means, they are sure to recur unless the conditions of paralysis and improper positions are removed.

WHY DEFORMITIES RECUR.

No matter how often the deformity may have been cured, if the paralysis still exists, there will be a tendency to a recurrence of the same shortening of certain muscles, with the same distortions as before, unless the positions are constantly secured by mechanical means. While the paralysis itself does not directly produce the unequal distribution of force, its existence renders the patient liable, from slight and accidental causes, to all those changes in the condition of the muscles which were discussed in the first part of this essay. In short, whatever may be the apparent hopelessness of the paralysis, the only object in treatment should be to remove it as far as possible, and in the carrying out of this idea the mechanical appliances can accomplish but the first step.

SPECIAL MEANS OF DEVELOPMENT.

The next thing to be attended to should be those means which directly tend to increase the nervous and muscular power of the affected member. And here we come back to the same remedies which are applicable in the first stages of the disease. We have labored long and patiently to imperfectly mend what, by proper management, might have been easily prevented, and now we begin our actual treatment. Our object is to increase the muscular power, and after the great and, to a certain extent, irreparable loss in time, we should be prepared to be satisfied vrith moderate amelioration, when if the means had been applied in time they might have gone far toward securing complete restoration. Still, the stimulating effect of heat and the gentle use of the muscles without over-taxing them seem to be the true physiological means for increasing their irritability and power.

And it is truly wonderful to what an extent the development may often be carried even in the worst cases. Indeed, there are few forms of distortion following infantile paralysis which are so bad that they can not be improved so as to afford the patient a serviceable limb. But it takes time and patience.

PARALYSIS OF UPPER EXTREMITIES.

Paralysis of the upper extremities is of frequent occurrence; and, incomprehensible as it would appear, on the theory that this form of paralysis arises from a lesion of the brain or spinal cord, in the larger number of cases, it is not accompanied by any paralysis of the lower portion of the body. There are cases of paralysis of the whole body and all extremities, or of one upper and one lower extremity. I have even seen a paralysis of the arm on one side accompanied with paralysis of the opposite leg! Yet in the majority of cases the paralysis affects only one upper extremity. The paralysis of an upper extremity is characterized by the same phenomena in all respects as when the disease affects a lower extremity. Wherever there is extension of a muscle, there we find the greatest weakness; and, on the other hand, wherever the muscles have been relaxed, then they have "contracted" or become shortened. From the nature of the case, the deltoid is apt to especially suffer. The weight of the whole arm makes continuous traction upon the deltoid, and we consequently find that muscle almost invariably extended and atrophied to the last degree–fig. 18. At the same time,

we are seldom troubled with serious muscular shortening, for the simple reason that the arm hangs in such a manner that no muscles are habitually relaxed; but all the muscles, both; the same, is relatively worse than of the lower extremities. There is seldom the same amount of paralysis in flexors and extensors, but the difference is generally that of different degrees of weakness, according as they have been subjected to different degrees of stretching. The obliteration of the deltoid and the stretching of the ligaments and separation of the head of the humerus from the glcnoid cavity is well shown in the cut.

Fig. 18.

flixors and extensors, are weakened by continuous stretching. For this reason, the paralysis of the arm, all other things being

The treatment for paralysis of the arm must be the same in principle as for paralysis in the lower extremities, with modifications corresponding to the form of injury to which it has been subjected since the paralysis occurred. As the arm has not become distorted by being bent down by the weight above it, we have comparatively few deformities, and these are not characterized by the same degree of alteration in the osseous forms as in the joints of the legs and feet. But we have other difficulties equally formidable. All the joints are partially drawn asunder, the articulating surfaces are smooth and rounded, and the muscles and ligaments are relaxed in many cases to the last degree.

THE MUSCLES MUST BE RELIEVED OF TRACTION.

There is one simple course to pursue. We must sustain the arm, and by thus relaxing the muscles, allow them to contract and regain somewhat of their impaired contractility. I have used with excellent effect a kind of sling that partially flexes the elbow, and sustains the whole arm so completely that the shoulder-joint is closed and the deltoid completely relaxed. To this can be attached suitable appliances for any deformities of the hand and fingers which may exist.

DEFORMITY OP HAND.

The principal or most common difficulty of the hand arises from atrophy of the adductor muscles of the thumb. By the atrophy of these muscles the thumb is drawn back into the same plane as the fingers, and the ability to adduct, flex, and oppose the other fingers and to grasp is entirely lost. The apparatus shown in fig. 19 is calculated to meet the difficulty. It is made of covered tin or zinc–gutta-percha will do–with the projection (a) to adduct and hold down the thumb; the

Fig. 19.

strap (5) keeps it in position. With the thumb thus held opposite the fingers, the patient at once begins to make the hand useful in grasping and holding objects. This new power also hastens the muscular development. The position of the thumb after atrophy of its adductors is well shown in fig. 18.

The sustaining of the arm in the sling must be continued uninterruptedly for a very long time–it will be of no use unless kept up without intermission–and should be combined with suitable exercise of the muscles as fast as they begin to recover contractile power. But six months suspension in the sling alone before the exercises were commenced would, in many cases, be good treatment.

The exercises should never consist of hanging or holding heavy substances; on the contrary, gentle and light exercises should be adapted to the feeble muscles.

HOW TO DETECT AND USE LATENT FORCE.

Fig. 20 shows an admirable apparatus for exercising the deltoid muscle. So long as the weight of the arm exceeds by the smallest fraction the strength of the muscle, it will continue to be overpowered and utterly in capable of causing the slightest movement of the arm. And yet there may be within it a latent strength, only needing opportunity to

Fig. 20.

be shown and developed till it might become adequate to effect ordinary movements. Suppose the arm weighs ten pounds, and the deltoid could lift but five pounds–how is this latent force to be made available? Simply by reducing the resistance to the muscle–that is, reducing the weight of the arm–to three or four pounds, or to any amount less tliiiu the capacity of the muscle, when we should immediately witness a movement of the arm by action of this muscle. The weight, "W, in the accompanying illustration, is moved to a point where it will just balance and neutralize so much of the weight of the arm as shall reduce the resistance to the capacity of the muscle. From this point we begin our development. As the strength of the muscle increases, less and less of the arm is balanced, till, by-and-by, the muscle becomes capable of raising the whole arm, and more. After that time the power in the muscle continues more than sufficient to accomplish motion. Other exercises, adapted to the action of the arm, forearm, wrist and fingers, must be employed, if we would have the development uniform. So of all actions of the various bodily members; apparatus must be contrived with such complete adaptability, that the natural action of the joint may be secured together with most delicate measure of muscular force.

Fig. 21.

Fig. 21 (like fig. 17, for the ankle) illustrates a lateral action at the knee. A rivet joint at A allows flexion and extension; the lateral motion at B is secured by the key

C, lengthening or shortening the side of the apparatus. In knock-knee, how-leg, and other deformities of the lower extremitie, lateral action is indispensable.

In what has been said, I have aimed to illustrate principles, and hence have shown the most simple adaptation of apparatus. And as regarding deformities, I have avoided extreme cases, and have confined my observations to such as, by following a consistent plan of treatment, may always reward our efforts with either cure or amelioration.

Conclusion.

The facts and arguments contained in the preceding pages may be summed up in the following propositions, viz.: 1. Infantile Paralysis is an arrest of vegetative development from some unknown cause.

2. The characteristics of this form of paralysis suggest a peripheric blight rather than a loss of central nerve-power.

3. With diminished nutrition, temperature and muscular power there is also diminished muscular irritability; and there is no such

thing as involuntary or reflex contraction in infantile paralysis.

4. The shortening of certain muscles is not a necessary consequence of infantile paralysis; and when it does occur, it is simply the adaptation of their length to the position they happen to be in.

5. It is entirely accidental which muscles become shortened, whether flexors or extensors.

6. Hence, deformities are not a necessary consequence of infantile paralysis, and when the are allowed to occur, the process of recovery is arrested.

7. When deformities have already formed, they should be treated for an ultimate end–viz., to bring the patient back to the place from which he should not have been allowed to diverge, where the treatment for s paralysis should begin.

8. Hence, tenotomy and mechanical appliances are only means to an end–the first steps of a course of treatment having in view the restoration of the muscular power.

9. The most natural means for this purpose is the supply of local heat–involving increased local circulation–together with local exercise corresponding with the position and ability of the part exercised.

10. The element of time must also be taken into consideration.

The following cases will still further elucidate the foregoing views:

Case 6.–T. T., aged two years and a half, was paralyzed while teething. Had had several attacks of sickness, but no diarrhoea; was nervous and feverish. After lying alternately in his crib and in his mothers arms for three days, he seemed convalescing, when, one day, on attempting to make him stand, it was discovered that the right leg was paralyzed. The next day his left arm was found to be also paralyzed. He at once began to improve, and in three weeks was able to push a chair about the room. In April, 18C2, seven mouths afterward, I saw him. He was then a very active, nervous boy, but plump, ruddy, and rather precocious. At that time the hand was useless, and he walked badly. After six weeks treatment the use of the arm and hand was fully restored. The leg and foot improved equally with the hand and arm. He had regained the use of the muscles, and could control all his motions; but he left before he had regained enough strength in the ankle to support his weight, and there was some shortening of the tendo-Achillis with diminished action of the flexors–not enough power to lift the foot. He wore no apparatus at that time, for I had not then learned to anticipate and provide for the effects of the weakened flexors. Two years afterward he returned with a fully formed talipes varus, and complete loss of power in the flexors of the foot. Efforts to extend the muscle proving unavailing, the tendo-Achillis was divided, in the fall of 1863. Returning home after the operation, I did not see him for several months, and when he came back, I found that extension of the muscle had been carried too far; the tendo-Achillis had been too much elongated. The result was, that the flexors of the foot had become in turn shortened and restored to active strength. Since then the chief treatment has been to reverse the effects of the too great lengthening of the tendo-Achillis–that is, to overcome the flexors and increase the strength of the gastrocnemius!

The points of special interest in this case are the paralysis of one arm and leg on opposite sides; the arrest of cure and the formation of talipes after recovery had gone on so far; and the transferring of the seat of shortened muscles from the posterior to the anterior side of the leg!

Case 7.–J. G., aged twelve years and five months. In March, 1865, had slight indisposition and loss of appetite, some fever, and headache occurring evening and morning, the latter increasing in severity as her strength diminished. Complained also of pain in the left leg. By the middle of April was much reduced, and had an attack of diptheria, from which she recovered in a few daj-s without any apparent change in the other symptoms. But from that time her previous unpleasant symptoms gradually lessened. She complained of pain in her back and legs, but gained in strength. About the first of June she began to try to walk; but there was found to be considerable shortening of the tendo-Achillis of the left heel. She tried crutches without avail, and finally could only creep a little upon her knees. I first saw her on the 20th of November following the attack. At that time there was paralysis of both logs, nearly complete loss of power in the left, and shortening of the flexors of the thighs and legs and of the extensors of the feet; the left foot particularly being extended nearly to a line with the leg. The extensors of the thighs and legs and the flexors of the feet were wholly powerless. All improvement which could have been of practical value had ceased, and she was apparently crippled for life. Believing that if the extended muscles could be speedily relieved, there would be a further effort of Nature to resume the repar-ative process (unfortunately interrupted by the progress of the deformities), my attention was at first directed to extending the shortened muscles. This was done by appropriate apparatus, and at the same time the muscles were brought into gentle use as fast as their action was made possible through liberating the motions. She at once began to improve, and in May following I had the satisfaction of seeing her walk erect and with the function of every muscle restored to her. The restoration is quite complete.

This case is related to illustrate the gradual and relatively prolonged course in the accession of the disease, as often happens in older patients, and also to show the fact, that even in a patient of her age it was not known at what time the paralysis occurred; the arrest of the recuperative process after the muscles were allowed to lose their dynamic relations; and the immediate resumption of recuperation when apparatus had restored them to their natural positions.

Case 8.–This case is only interesting in consideration of the wide extent and completeness of the paralysis in connection with the mild character of her symptoms; and also, that even in so grave a case improvement is still steadily going on, though at a very slow rate.

S. W., aged seven years, complained of some slight indisposition for two or three days; she had some fever, and headache. A physician was called, who pronounced the symptoms of a typhoid character, and in a day or two she was found to be completely paralyzed from head to foot. This was in August, 1864. I saw her in May, 1865. At that time she had regained tolerable use of one hand; but could neither stand nor sit, and the so-called contractions existed wherever circumstances had favored their occurrence. Of course the power of their antagonists was entirely gone. By proper apparatus the deformities were reduced, the contractions overcome, and, as before stated, she has from that day steadily continued to gain. Although she can not yet walk, no deformity has occurred, nor can occur so long as the same principles of treatment are carried out.

Case 9.–The interesting feature in the following case is the good degree of improvement in the muscular power as a direct result of the simple extension of the contracted muscles. The development of muscle would without doubt have been much greater if her treatment had also embraced the local exercises; but in that case it would not have so well illustrated the views so often insisted on in these pages, that improvement is arrested long before it has reached its ultimate limit by positions which allow of a shortening of muscles; and also, that sometimes, as in this case, the process of recovery may be resumed and carried forward to a considerable extent years afterward, if the injured muscles are relieved by extending the shortened ones. In this case there was no power in the flexors of the foot and extensors of the leg during eight years; but they immediately regained a considerable degree of strength when the cause of the suspension of improvement was removed. Apparatus, shown in figs. 12 and 13, were furnished, with appropriate directions. As I had never seen the case but twice, and it had received no other treatment, I wrote to the father for the facts, which may as well be given in his own words:

"My daughter Josie, who was placed under your care in May and November, 1865, and has at home followed your directions in wearing more or less apparatus adjusted to her partially paralyzed leg, first manifested to us that her leg was debilitated when about eighteen months of age. She walked when about a year old, then gave up walking. We attributed the fact to debility from teething. When she resumed walking, at about eighteen months of age, the weakness in one leg was discovered. We flattered ourselves she would outgrow it, having no suspicion of the real trouble. Her condition when you saw her in May, 1865, you can describe better than I can. She was then nine years and nine months old. I can describe no symptoms except weakness in the leg; wasting of the flesh, reducing it to from one to one and a half inches in circumference below the size of the other; a constant liability to fall upon that knee, so much so that a pad was kept on it to prevent bruising; an entire inability to go either up or down stairs by placing the weak foot or leg before, the other. She also uniformly bore her weight on the other leg, and thus distorted her form. When she went to you, she could bear her weight on that leg alone, but was powerless in the effort to kick with it, or to throw her foot in front without throwing out the whole limb, and could not approach toward a hop upon it.

"She has since that time shown much improvement, sufficient to afford me much encouragement. She can hop on it feebly, raising herself by a hop on that foot about three inches perpendicularly without difficulty; can throw out her foot in front, but not with much energy. Her lameness is still quite perceptible in walking, and still more so when running. She falls but seldom; her limb shows more hardness of muscle and fullness. The apparent projection of the knee-pan has to some extent diminished.

"Yours, J. M."